THE ORIGINAL KETO DIET BOOK

Lose Weight Eating Healthy and Tasty incl. Meal Prep Special (UK version)

Marc J. Williams

TABLE OF CONTENTS

Introduction

Most people strive to adopt a healthy lifestyle by cautiously choosing what they eat and watching their weight. For this reason, quite a number of individuals are leveraging on the new low carb and high-fat diet so that they can lose weight consistently. Eating the right food helps reduce lifestyle diseases, gives you more energy, and improves your mental health. On this account, we have put together a simple but comprehensive Keto Book, to help you not only lose weight but also eat healthily and enjoy tasty meals.

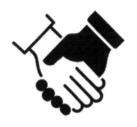

How Is Your Body Likely to React to The Keto Diet?

Initially, your body may experience Keto flu. It's a carbohydrate withdrawal symptom that has the symptoms of fatigue, headache, mood swings, insomnia, and irritability. You may also experience brain fog that occurs when your body reacts to the energy level changes. The reduction in insulin level due to an abrupt change from carbs to fats results in a diuretic effect. Some individuals also experience high levels of dehydration than normal.

Experiencing Keto Flu does not mean that you should stop dieting. All you need is to drink lots of water, eat more salt, and increase your potassium intake.

- ✓ Your body may also react to the Keto diet in the following ways:
- ✓ Your insulin sensitivity will improve
- ✓ You may have muscle cramps
- ✓ Your breath can smell
- ✓ You may have increased energy levels
- ✓ Inflammation may be greatly reduced.

Does Keto Help Build Muscle?

Yes, Keto is very important in muscle building. However, there are misguided ideas that may discourage you from getting started on the Keto diet. The misconception is that you need carbohydrates to build muscles. A Keto diet will help in building muscles just like a high carb diet. The benefit of building muscles using a Keto diet is that you will not accumulate fat.

To build muscles with Keto you need to eat more calories, train your muscles regularly, eat minimal carbohydrates and enough proteins, and have supplements that will give you more energy levels

Is Keto Diet Healthy and Safe?

The Keto diet is generally safe. Studies show that it doesn't expose you to any danger and is recommendable for obese and overweight individuals. It is advisable to, however, consult your physician when trying out a new weight loss plan or new diet. If you are pregnant, breastfeeding, have underlying conditions like blood pressure or you are using insulin, a Keto diet will not be ideal.

You should also take into account your physical activity. Always go on a Keto diet when your level of activity is low. To be safe and ensure enough energy levels, always use fats for more energy requirements, drink lots of water, only eat when you feel hungry, focus on whole foods, exercise more, and reduce your overall protein intake.

How Long Can One Diet When On the Keto Diet?

One can take the diet for as long as they enjoy it. If you feel healthier, energetic and your physician recommends that you continue, you can enjoy the diet. You don't need to continue with your previous way of eating. Keto, as experts say is no longer a diet but a lifestyle that many people are happy to adopt.

How Much Weight Can You Lose On the Keto Diet?

After following your Keto Diet for a week, you are most likely to see some weight loss results. Most people lose between two to ten pounds. Most of this weight loss is actually water weight because most of the carbohydrates stored in your body retain water.

Our bodies store carbohydrates in form of glycogen which contains water. If you reduce your intake of carbs the body loses the glycogen plus the water retained. Your first week of Keto diet will mostly be water since the body has not stored carbohydrates. When you burn the glycogen stored, the body uses fat as energy.

Can I Drink Alcohol While On the Keto Diet?

You can drink alcohol while dieting. Drinking does not affect the process of Ketosis. You should however avoid wine and beer. This is because they contain grains, sugar, and a high number of carbs. You can also opt for alcohol that does not contain any syrups, sugars, and added flavors.

You should, however, know that while on a Keto diet, drinking can have more hangovers than normal. Alcohol can also awaken your cravings and it may be difficult to avoid non-Keto foods.

Types of Keto Diets: Which One Is Best for You

A ketogenic diet is meant to cause ketosis; where body fat is broken into ketones. Your body will therefore get energy from ketones and not glucose.

There are many different types of ketogenic diets, we will explain the five different types so that you can identify the one that is best for you.

Standard Ketogenic Diet (SKD)

This diet is simple and very common. Many people find it very easy to follow. It consists of very low carbs, high fat diet, and moderate portions of protein. The fat is around 75 percent.

Your daily consumption of a ketogenic diet can be:

- ✓ 50g carbohydrate
- ✓ 60g protein
- ✓ Any amount of fat

Cyclical Ketogenic Diet (CKD)

Also referred to as carb backloading, you can have more carbs during some days then have other days of higher carbs.

This diet is ideal for highly active persons like athletes who use high carbohydrates to replace the glucose lost during workouts.

Targeted Ketogenic Diet (TKD)

This diet is similar to the standard ketogenic diet. However, carbohydrates can be consumed during times of great exercise. You can therefore consume any amount of carbohydrate as long as you exercise.

In this diet, the carbohydrates you consume before a physical exercise or after will often be burnt down efficiently. Our muscles need an increase in energy when we are active.

High Protein Ketogenic Diet

This diet is a high protein diet than other diets. It has 60% fat, 5% carbohydrates, and 35% protein.

Research shows that a high protein diet is ideal for weight loss. However, it is not clear if there are long term health implications if the diet is adopted for many years.

Calorie-Restricted Ketogenic Diet

In this diet, the calorie intake is greatly reduced. Research has proven that ketogenic diets are successful regardless of a calorie intake restriction. This is because ketosis and eating fat prevent one from eating large portions that can result in weight gain.

The Benefits of the Keto Diet

The keto diet is very popular for the health benefits it offers. It's not only beneficial for this but also for other advantages gained. Keto is therefore more of a lifestyle and not just a diet.

Here are the benefits of the Keto diet.

Weight Loss

The ketogenic diet is very efficient in weight loss. It helps in reducing appetite and boosting metabolism. It fills you up and reduces hunger causing hormones. Strict adherence to a Keto diet reduces your appetite hence promoting your weight loss.

A 2013 study reveals that people who followed the Keto diet lost 2 pounds compared to those following a low-fat diet. A Keto diet is therefore your ideal weight loss plan.

Reduces Certain Cancers

Studies show that the diet is a safe and very suitable complementary treatment that can be used for radiation therapy and chemotherapy for certain cancers. This is because it causes more oxidative stress in the cancer cells compared to normal cells hence causing them to die.

A 2018 study shows that ketogenic diets help in reducing blood sugar, which lowers the danger of insulin complications.

May Protect Brain Function

According to studies, ketones generated during the Keto diet offer neuroprotective benefits that protect and strengthen nerve and brain cells.

A Keto diet may therefore help a person manage and prevent conditions like Alzheimer's disease.

Helps Fight Type-2 Diabetes

People with type-2 diabetes often have increased insulin production. The ketogenic diet removes the sugar from one's diet. It also lowers the HbA1c count which reverses type-2 diabetes.

Following a Ketogenic diet reduces the key markers that cause type-2 diabetes.

Increased Energy

Our body stores a lot of glycogen which needs to be refueled to maintain energy levels. Your body, however, has plenty of fats that have already been stored, which means that in ketosis there is an energy source that will not run out.

With a Keto diet, you will have more enough the whole day.

How to Start the Keto Diet?

Step 1: Be Stress-Free and Halt Tasking Duties

Choose a week that that requires very little physical exercise from you. Ensure you do not have dinner plans, birthday parties, or dates. Don't start your diet when you are traveling. It is important to ensure that your family is also aware so that they can offer you their support without judgment.

Step 2: Clean Out Your Refrigerator and Pantry.

Ensure that your kitchen does not have non-ketogenic food which you'll be tempted to try them out. It's best if you removed everything out. You can share junk foods with friends and relatives who exercise vigorously.

Step 3: Restock with Ketogenic Foods

To get on the right track, stock all the ketogenic foods you will need. Get a meal plan, ingredients, and the food list that will guide you. You'll definitely spend money on your journey to fitness. Your investment will be worth it in the long run since you will be more vibrant and play more with your loved ones.

Step 4: Decide On the Meals to Skip

You need to decide which meal you will skip in a day. You may prefer to skip your breakfast in order to have the mental energy for your day's work, lunch, or dinner. Deciding which meal to skip helps you stick to a daily routine throughout your diet.

Step 5: Reduce Carbs and Increase Proteins and Fats

During your first week, you need to reduce the number of carbs you consume. Eating the right amount of fats, proteins, and carbs helps you quickly get into ketosis.

You can always adjust your meal plan by adding proteins and fats to your meal. You can always eat plenty of avocado, eggs and coconut oil, sardines, and olive oil.

Step 6: Start Your Day with A Ketone-Boosting Routine

To start your Keto diet, you need to drink a glass of water in the morning. This will ensure the water stored in your body is less and more carbs burnt. You can also take coconut oil as an energy supplement.

Step 7: Track Your Ketone Levels

The ketogenic diet gets your body to burn fats instead of glucose. You need to check your ketone levels using a blood ketone tracker. Tracking your level is important in helping you know if you are on track or when something is not right.

How Much Does the Keto Plan Cost

One good thing with ketogenic diets is that they can be free. There are countless free online resources, therefore, there is no need to buy products that offer instant ketosis. If you do not consume carbohydrates, your body will automatically undergo ketosis without many resources.

How Can You Prepare for a Cheap Keto Diet?

There are several ways you can reduce your grocery budget and save money in the long run. Here are ways to ensure you have a cheap Keto Diet

Get ready to engage in pantry cooking, leftovers, and cheap Keto meals

Invest in cheap healthy meals. You can opt for the garden salad, vegetables, and meat. Ensure that the ingredients are easily available and not costly.

Utilize the leftovers in making meals; making a new meal while preparing another meal is costly. One meal that is eaten now and frozen for later cuts down on your budget.

You can also cook what you have in stock other than always buying ingredients every time you need to cook a meal.

Choose cheap cuts of meat, shop weekly, and buy meat in bulk

Buying chicken pieces as opposed to the whole chicken can be cheaper. You can also save by buying ground beef, steak, and pork chops. Shopping weekly is cheap. You can get sales on different meats or chicken. Designing your weekly meal plan will save you a lot of money. When you buy in excess, you can always freeze the meat that has been bought in bulk.

Save on vegetables and fruits

You can save by buying the fruits that are in season, have a small garden where you can have your fruits and vegetables, or shop at a farmer's garden.

Buy groceries in online stores

Buying your groceries online reduces the temptation of buying other things on impulse and inflating your budget.

Other ways of reducing your Keto diet are; ensure you buy in bulk, check for discounts on selected oils, and buy on selected stores that are always lower than the rest.

What to Eat On the Keto Diet?

A ketogenic diet limits the number of carbs consumed daily to between 20g and 50g. Many foods that are of fat and protein content can fit into this category.

Here is a list of the foods you can eat while on a Keto diet:

Vegetables

Vegetables have low carbs and calories. They contain high amounts of nutrients such as vitamin C and other minerals. Vegetables are also high in fiber which is not absorbed and digested like carbs. Always look for the net carb count which is the total amount of carbohydrates less fiber content.

Vegetables have less net carbs. When you consume a serving of starchy vegetables such as yam, beets, and potatoes, you may be over your daily total carb limit. Non-starchy vegetables such as raw spinach and cooked Brussels sprouts contain less than 1g of carb. Other vegetables such as cauliflower, broccoli, and kale help in reducing the high risks associated with a heart attack and cancer.

Cheese

Cheese is delicious and very nutritious. There are however different types of cheese. Many of these varieties are low in carbs and high in fat content. This makes them ideal for a Keto diet. 28g of cheddar cheese contains 7g protein and 1g carbs. Though high in fats, cheese does not expose one to the risk of a heart attack. Eating cheese regularly reduces the loss of muscle and energy that happens as one comes of age.

Avocados

Avocados are very healthy and ideal for the keto diet. 100g of avocado contains a total of 9g carbs. It also contains minerals and vitamins such as potassium which are important. The high potassium levels in avocadoes make the keto diet very easy to transition. You also get improved triglyceride and cholesterol levels.

Meat and Poultry

Meat and poultry do not have any carbs and are very rich in vitamins and minerals such as zinc, selenium, and potassium. They also have high protein levels that preserve mass when one is on a low carb diet. One needs to eat grass-fed meat. Such meat has antioxidants, conjugated linoleic acid, and omega-3 fats. On the other hand, grain-fed animals do not contain such nutrients.

Eggs

One egg contains 1g of carbohydrates and less than 6g protein. Eggs are therefore ideal for a ketogenic diet. They also help you to feel more full since they trigger those hormones. Your blood sugar level will be more stable leading to lower calorie intake. Egg yolks have a high cholesterol level but they do not raise blood levels. Your risks of heart disease are reduced when you eat eggs.

Other foods that you can take on a keto diet include, nuts and seeds, plain yogurt, olive oil, coconut oil, berries, butter and cream, olives, unsweetened tea and coffee, dark chocolate, and cocoa butter

Foods That Should Not Be Eaten When On the Keto Diet

Cake

All types of cakes have a lot of carbs and are not advised when on a Keto diet. They also contain high levels of sugar that destroy insulin levels and ruin the process of Ketosis.

Milk

All kinds of milk are not to be taken on a Keto diet. This is because milk has high levels of milk sugar and lactose. A serving of milk provides 12g sugar.

Apples

Many natural fruits just like apples contain high levels of carbohydrates. Eating an apple equals a total intake of 20g in your body. That level is equivalent to the total number of daily carb intake allowed in a Keto diet.

Bananas

Bananas have a high percentage of calories. One banana gives you a total of 24g of carbohydrates. It also contains sugar which inhibits your body in getting into Ketosis.

Grapes

Grapes are other types of healthy fruit that should be avoided when on a Keto diet. They contain a lot of sugars; a 100g serving gives you 22g carbohydrates. You can however eat blueberries and raspberries that have low carbs.

RECIPES

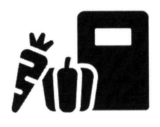

Breakfast Recipes

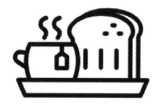

Keto Feta Quiche and Spinach

Time: 55 minutes | Servings 8
Kcal 234, Carbs 2.7g/0.09oz, Fats 20.2g/0.71oz, Proteins 9.4g/0.33oz, Fiber 1g/0.03oz

Ingredients:

- 🍽 23g/¼ cup of parmesan cheese

- 🍽 2g/½ a teaspoon of garlic powder

- 🍽 14g/1 tablespoon of butter

- 🍽 4g/1 teaspoon of onion powder

- 🍽 4 eggs

- 🍽 A pinch of salt

- 🍽 240ml/1 cup of heavy whipping cream

- 🍽 A pinch of pepper

- 🍽 57g/½ cup of grated mozzarella

- 🍽 250g/1 packet of frozen spinach (thawed and drained)

- 🍽 100g/⅔ cup of crumbled feta cheese

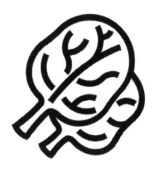

Instructions:

1. Bring the oven to a temperature of 180 °C/ 355 °F on a conventional oven, or 160 °C/ 320 °F using the fan-assisted version.

2. Now apply a generous amount of butter on a 25cm/8-inch baking dish.

3. Crack the eggs in a separate mixing bowl and whisk evenly.

4. Add in the seasonings, half of the grated mozzarella cheese, and the parmesan cheese to the whisked eggs.

5. Drain and squeeze as much moisture from the spinach before scattering on the pre-greased baking dish.

6. Reduce the feta into smaller chunks and add on top of the spinach.

7. Now empty the egg mixture on over before topping with the remainder of the mozzarella cheese.

8. Put in the oven and allow cooking for 45 minutes till nice and cooked.

9. Allow cooling for a few minutes then go ahead and slice.

Keto Single-Serve Peach Cobbler

Time: 35 minutes | Servings 4
Kcal 273, Carbs 7.3g/0.26oz, Fats 24.8g/0.9oz, Proteins 6g/0.21oz, Fiber 3.4g/0.12oz

Ingredients:

- 28g/1oz of virgin coconut oil or unsalted butter
- 225g/8oz of sliced peaches. (Stoned removed)
- 15ml/1 tablespoon of fresh lime juice or lemon
- 20g/0.7oz of brown sugar
- 1g/¼ teaspoon of nutmeg
- 1g/¼ teaspoon of cinnamon
- Topping
- 28g/1oz of virgin coconut oil or unsalted butter
- 100g/3.5oz of almond flour
- 20g/0.7oz of brown sugar

Instructions:

1. Bring the oven to a temperature of 220 °C/ 425 °F on a conventional oven or 200 °C/ 400 °F in a fan assisted variation.

2. Put equal peach slices into 4 single cup ramekins.

3. Spread atop with some brown sugar and cinnamon.

4. Now drizzle with some lime plus the 200g coconut oil or butter.

5. Cook in the oven for 20 minutes mixing midway through for even cooking.

6. While the peach is baking, add the remaining butter, sugar, and almond flour into a separate mixing bowl and whisk thoroughly into a dough.

7. Once the peach is nice and soft, put the dough crumbles on atop and allow them to bake for 5 more minutes

8. After 5 minutes, take out of the oven before cooling shortly.

9. Alternatively, you could dust with some ground sugar which will make the cobbler crisp up during cooking.

Spinach and Feta ShakShuka

Time: 20 minutes | Servings 2

Kcal 510, Carbs 9g/0.32oz, Fats 42.8g/1.5oz, Proteins 19.5g/0.69oz, Fiber 4.3g/0.15oz

Ingredients:

- 🍽 30ml/2 tablespoons of extra virgin olive oil
- 🍽 30ml/2 tablespoons of avocado oil or ghee
- 🍽 38g/1.3oz of crumbled feta cheese
- 🍽 ½ chopped and sliced yellow onions
- 🍽 4 eggs
- 🍽 1 clove of minced garlic
- 🍽 200g/7oz of fresh spinach
- 🍽 1 small sliced red bell pepper onion
- 🍽 A pinch of salt
- 🍽 60g/4 tablespoons of tomato paste
- 🍽 2g/½ a teaspoon of ground Turmeric
- 🍽 A pinch of black pepper

- 🍽 120ml/½ a cup of water or chicken stalk
- 🍽 4g/1 teaspoon of ground cumin

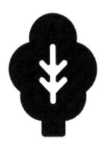

Instructions:

1. Clean and drain the spinach before cutting off the crunchy stalk. Coarsely, slice the spinach leaves and chop the stalks into small pieces.

2. Generously, grease a skillet using butter or avocado oil and heat up over medium temperatures.

3. Begin by putting in the onions and let them cook for 3 minutes before adding in the minced garlic and cooking for another minute.

4. Once done, put in the chopped bell peppers and spinach stalks and cook for 5 minutes till tender yet crispy.

5. Pour in the chicken stock or water and allow the mixture to simmer.

6. Top with the seasoning (salt, pepper, turmeric, and cumin) before adding in the spinach. Let them cook roughly for a minute till nice and wilted.

7. Create 4 circular wells then crack an egg in each well.

8. Bring the heat down then cover the pan. Allow cooking for 5 minutes till egg whites gets almost set but the yolk remains runny.

9. Now sprinkle atop with some crumbled feta and cook for another minute.

10. Top with olive oil and a garnish of your choice.

11. Serve and enjoy while warm.

The Keto Tuna ShakShuka

Time: 20 minutes | Serving 3

Kcal 438, Carbs 4g/0.14oz, Fats 33.4g/1.18oz, Proteins 29.8g/1.05oz, Fiber 1.1g/0.03oz

Ingredients:

- A pinch of sea salt
- A pinch of pepper
- 20ml/2 tablespoons of extra virgin olive oil
- 30ml/2 tablespoons of extra virgin avocado oil or ghee
- ½ chopped yellow onion
- 6 eggs
- 2 cloves of diced garlic
- 30g/2 tablespoons of chopped cilantro

- 30g/2 tablespoons of tomato paste
- 255g/9oz of drained tuna (Canned)
- 240ml/½ a cup of brine from tuna
- 4g/1teaspoon of turmeric
- 2g/½ a teaspoon of paprika
- 2g/ ½ a teaspoon of ground cumin

Instructions:

1. Generously grease the inside of a skillet using avocado oil.

2. For 5 minutes, sauté the onions before putting in the diced garlic. Allow cooking for a minute.

3. Once everything is nice and fragrant, add in the tomato paste and cook for 1 minute. Now add in the tuna and mix well.

4. Put in salt, pepper, water and all the spices then stir.

5. Allow the mixture to boil before bringing down the heat to a medium and let the food simmer till nice and thick.

6. Top with some chopped cilantro then stir.

7. Create 6 wells and crack an egg in each well.

8. Let the egg whites cook partially before covering to cook the top part of the eggs. Don't let the yolk overcook.

9. Alternatively, sprinkle with some cheddar cheese and cook some more.

10. Garnish with cilantro before serving.

Keto Apricot Crumble Coffee Cake

Time: 75 minutes | Servings 10
Kcal 306, Carbs 6.4g/0,22oz, Fats 25.9g/0.91oz, Proteins 10.9g/ 0.38oz, Fiber 3.7g/0.13oz

Ingredients:

- 6 apricots with stones removed
- 200g/7.1oz of almond flour
- 4 large separated eggs
- 30g/1.1oz coconut flour
- 150g/¾ a cup of granulated sweetener
- 25g/0.9oz egg white protein powder
- 1 stick (113g/4oz) of softened unsalted butter
- 8g/2 teaspoon of gluten-free baking powder
- 10ml/2 teaspoon of sugar-free vanilla extract
- Zest of 1 organic lemon
- For the topping
- 50g/1.8oz almond flour

- 10g/0.4oz of granulated low-carb sweetener
- 15g/1 tablespoon of unsalted butter

Instructions:

1. Bring the oven to a temperature of 170 °C/ 340 °F.

2. To prepare the cake base, combine the almond flour, sweetener, egg white proteins powder, and the zest in a bowl and mix well.

3. Separate the yolk from the whites. Using a different bowl, cream the butter and the sweetener using a hand mixture.

4. Add in the yolks and vanilla extract and process till even.

5. In another bowl, mix the egg whites till soft peaks appear.

6. Combine ⅓ of the flour dry mixture into the egg mixture carefully. Add in the remainder in two portions and mix thoroughly.

7. Finish by folding in the fluffy egg whites in three portions.

8. Now using a round springform pan lined with parchment paper, transfer in all the batter.

9. Arrange the apricots on the batter having the cut side down.

10. Put into the oven and cook for 45 minutes till the cake is set and the top is golden brown.

11. While the cake base is baking, combine the remainder of the almond flour, sweetener, and butter into a mixing bowl and carefully combine to cookie dough.

12. Remove the cake base from the oven before topping with the crumbled cookie dough and bake for an additional 8 minutes.

13. Allow cooling before removing from the pan.

14. Slice and enjoy!

Keto Strawberry Ginger Crumble

Time: 45minutes | 8 Servings

Kcal 230, Carbs 6.7g/0.24oz, Fats 19.7g/0.7oz, Proteins 5.2g/0.18oz, Fiber 4.5g/0.16oz

Ingredients:

- 🍽 A generous pinch of sea salt
- 🍽 24g/2 tablespoons of chia seeds
- 🍽 550g/20oz of fresh strawberries (halved)
- 🍽 2g/½ a teaspoon of vanilla powder
- 🍽 4g/½ a teaspoon of ginger powder
- 🍽 4g/1 teaspoon of cinnamon
- 🍽 45g/3 tablespoons of unsalted ghee or coconut oil
- 🍽 50g/ ¼ cup of granulated low carb sweetener
- 🍽 For the topping
- 🍽 45g/3 tablespoons of unsalted ghee, butter, or coconut oil
- 🍽 150g/1½ cups of almond flour
- 🍽 30g/1.1oz of low carb sweetener

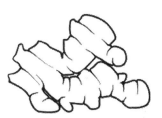

Instructions:

1. Bring the oven to a temperature of 195 °C/ 380 °F.

2. Slice the strawberries into halves and chop the ginger into fine pieces.

3. On a baking dish, place the halved berries and ginger. Add in ¼ cup sweetener, butter, cinnamon, and vanilla.

4. Combine everything by tossing before allowing to bake in the oven for 15 minutes, tossing halfway done.

5. Once done, remove from the oven, top with some chia seed before combining everything together, and set aside for 15 minutes.

6. In the meantime, combine the remaining butter, almond flour, and sweetener in a bowl and combine using your hands till you achieve a thick dough.

7. Spread the crumbled dough over the strawberries and put back into the oven for 10 minutes till the topping turns slightly golden.

8. Serve and enjoy when cool.

Keto Chocolate Pancake Cereal

Time: 15 minutes | Servings 4
Kcal 248, Carbs 4.1g/0.14oz, Fats 20.6g/0.73oz, Proteins 10.1g/0.36oz, Fiber 5.3g/0.18oz

Ingredients:

- 🍽 4 large eggs

- 🍽 30g/¼ a cup of coconut flour

- 🍽 45ml/3 tablespoons of melted virgin coconut oil

- 🍽 43g/½ a cup of cacao powder

- 🍽 60ml/ ¼ cup of unsweetened coconut yogurt

- 🍽 2g/ ½ a teaspoon gluten-free baking powder

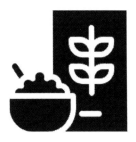

Instructions:

1. Collect, assemble, and weigh all the ingredients.

2. Now combine all the dry ingredients in a single mixing bowl and mix thoroughly.

3. In a second bowl, combine 1 tablespoon of coconut oil with yogurt and the eggs. Mix well and pour into the dry ingredient mixture.

4. Mix into a nice smooth batter.

5. Release all the batter into a piping bottle.

6. Using medium heat, bring a skillet to heat up.

7. Generously coat the insides of the skillet with the remaining coconut oil.

8. Squeeze the pancakes into small 2cm/ ¾-inches circles on the skillet.

9. For approximately a minute, cook the pancakes before flipping to the other side.

10. Remember to grease the pan in between batches.

11. Serve with topping of your choice.

Avocado Bacon Frittata

Time: 35 minutes | Serves 4
Kcal 467, Carbs 7g/0.24oz, Fat 38g/1.3oz, Protein 22g/ 0.77oz, Fiber 5g/0.17oz

Ingredients:

- Finely chopped red chili

- 6 beaten eggs

- Full avocado; peeled, stoned and chopped into fairly large pieces

- 12 halved baby plum tomatoes

- 200g/7oz bag mixed salad leaves

- 8 rasher smoked bacon

- 4g/A teaspoon of Dijon mustard

- 45ml/3 tablespoon olive oil

- 10ml/2 teaspoon red wine vinegar

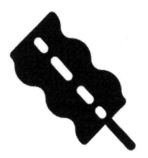

Instructions:

1. Preheat an ovenproof nonstick pan.

2. Fry the rashers in high heat till brown and crispy.

3. When cooked, make two batches of four each.

4. Chop one batch and break the other into large pieces and clean the pan.

5. Bring the grill to heat and warm a tablespoon of oil in a pan.

6. Season the egg and put in the chopped bacon then pour into the pan.

7. Cook for about 8 minutes on medium to low heat until it sets.

8. Carefully arrange the chopped avocado pieces and remaining bacon on top and grill for 3 minutes.

9. Mix the chili, mustard, and vinegar in the remaining oil.

10. Throw in the tomatoes and salad leaves.

11. Finally, make 4 frittata wedges and serve.

Halloumi, Cabbage, and Pesto Breakfast Hash

Time: 15 minutes | Servings 2
Kcal 682, Carbs 7.2g/0.25oz, Fats 61g/2.15oz, Proteins 25g/0.88oz, Fiber 5.2g/0.18oz

Ingredients:

- 45g/3 tablespoons of pestos
- 45ml/3 tablespoons of divided extra virgin coconut oil or olive oil
- 2 large eggs
- 300g/10.6oz ½ head savoy or green cabbage
- 150g/5.3oz of halloumi
- Cracked pepper for serving

Instructions:

1. Remove the outer leaves and set aside. Cut all the inner thick pieces if you are using the savoy cabbage.

2. Carefully chop the cabbage into ribbons

3. Pour 1 tablespoon of oil into a good-sized frying pan before heating under medium heat.

4. Put in the cabbage and cook for 5 minutes tossing occasionally till the cabbage softens. If you are using green cabbage, it will cook slightly longer than the savoy cabbage.

5. Reduce the halloumi into 1½ cm/½-inch cubes.

6. Using a different pan, pour another tablespoon of oil and put it in the halloumi cubes.

7. Using medium heat, let the halloumi cubes cook till both sides brown evenly.

8. Now transfer the cooked halloumi into the pan with cabbages before adding in the pesto and mix thoroughly.

9. Use low heat to cook the mixture.

10. Finally, add the remainder of the oil to the pan you cooked the halloumi in and bring it to heat.

11. Crack in the eggs and cook till the egg whites begin to set. Be sure not to overcook the eggs.

12. Serve by dividing the cabbage into two plates and topping with an egg in each plate.

13. Sprinkle with the cracked pepper and enjoy.

Low Carb Green Omelet

Time: 15 minutes | Servings 2
Kcal 528, Carbs 3.8g/0.13oz, Fats 41.9g/1.48oz, Proteins 30.9g/1.08oz, Fiber 4.2g/0.15oz

Ingredients:

For the omelet

- 🍽 30ml/2 tablespoons of extra virgin olive oil
- 🍽 4 large eggs
- 🍽 60g/2.1oz of fresh spinach
- 🍽 Pepper and salt
- 🍽 30g/¼ cup of loosely packed parsley
- 🍽 80ml/⅓ a cup of unsweetened almond milk
- 🍽 30g/⅓ a cup of grated parmesan cheese

For the fillings

- 🍽 80g/2.8oz of smoked salmon
- 🍽 ½ large sliced avocado
- 🍽 30g/¼ cup of loosely packed parsley
- 🍽 50 g/1.8oz crumbled feta

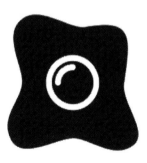

Instructions:

1. Begin by combining in all the omelet ingredients and the eggs in a food processor. Purse thoroughly till the spinach is finely chopped and well combined.

2. Using a good-sized pan, bring some oil to heat and pour in half of the omelet mixture and swirl to cover the base of the pan.

3. Allow the omelet to cook for 2 minutes or until it begins to set. Now, to one half of the omelet, top with some feta, avocado, parsley, and salmon then fold and cook for 2 more minutes.

4. Do the same with the remainder of the omelet mixture.

5. Serve and enjoy while warm

Lunch Recipes

Low-Carb Palmini Spaghetti Bolognese

Time: 20 minutes | Servings 4
Kcal 474, Carbs 6.3g/0.22oz, Fats 37.2g/1.31oz, Proteins 25.3g/0.89oz, Fiber 4.1g/0.14oz

Ingredients:

- 500g/1.1 lb ground beef
- 450g/ 1 lb palmini linguine noodles (2 cans)
- 300ml/1¼ a cup of homemade marinara sauce
- 15g/1 tablespoon of grated parmesan cheese
- Some chopped basil for garnish

Instructions:

1. Remove the palmini from the cans and drain using a colander.
2. Rinse over running water before setting aside.
3. Now, put the ground beef in a nonstick skillet and cook over medium to high heat till nice and brown for roughly 10 minutes.
4. Pour in the marinara sauce and stir through evenly.
5. On a serving dish, place half the marinara ground beef and top with the noodles. You could warm the noodles in a microwave or serve it like that.
6. Finally, top with some grated parmesan and basil.
7. Enjoy!

Keto Chicken Spinach and Artichoke Casserole

Time: 60 minutes | Servings 6
Kcal 499, Carbs 6.7g/0.24oz, Fats 31.5g/1.11oz, Proteins 43g/1.51oz, Fiber 4.9g/0.17oz

Ingredients:

- 23g/0.8oz of finely grated Parmesan
- 30ml/2 tablespoons of butter or ghee
- 115g/1 cup of shredded mozzarella
- 1kg/2.2 lbs Of skinless and boneless chicken thighs
- Pepper and salt
- 250g/8.8oz of frozen spinach (drained and defrosted)
- 8g/2 teaspoons of onion powder
- 400g/14.1oz of artichoke hearts (1 can)
- 1 clove of minced garlic
- 110g/½ a cup of paleo mayonnaise
- 63g/¼ cup of Greek yogurt

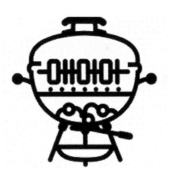

Instructions:

1. Using a conventional oven preheat to 200 °C/ 400 °F, or 180 °C/ 355 °F on the fan-assisted version.

2. Generously grease a good-sized baking dish with ghee or butter.

3. On a single layer, arrange the chicken thigh pieces on the baking sheet. (Be sure to defrost and drain excess water if you are using a frozen chicken)

4. Chop the artichokes and garlic finely using a knife or a small food processor.

5. Transfer the chopped artichokes and garlic into a mixing bowl and add in the spices, mayo, and yogurt then mix thoroughly.

6. Drain excess moisture from the spinach, put in the artichoke mixture, and mix well.

7. When evenly mixed, put in ⅔ of the grated Parmesan cheese and mix further.

8. Now, empty the mixture atop the chicken thigh pieces and sprinkle the remainder of the cheese on top.

9. Cook in the oven for 45 minutes till brown and well cooked.

10. Serve and enjoy while warm.

Low-Carb Crispy Fried KFC Chicken

Time: 25 minutes | Servings 8 pieces
Kcal 463, Carbs 1.8g/0.06oz, Fats 32.7g/1.15oz, Proteins 39.3g/1.39oz, Fiber 0.6g/0.02oz

Ingredients:

Dry

- 75g/2.7oz of unsweetened whey protein powder
- 6g/1½ teaspoon of paprika
- 1g/¼ a teaspoon of cracked black pepper
- 2g/½ a teaspoon of dried thyme
- 4g/1 teaspoon of sea salt
- 4g/1 teaspoon of garlic powder
- 2g/½ a teaspoon of dried oregano
- 1g/¼ teaspoon of cayenne pepper

Wet

- ½ a teaspoon of Dijon mustard
- 1 egg
- 1 teaspoon of sriracha hot sauce
- 15ml/1 tablespoon of heavy whipping cream
- 400g/14.1oz chicken fillets
- Enough oil for deep frying

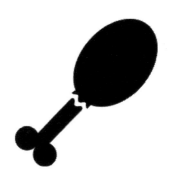

Instructions:

1. In a mixing bowl, add in the pepper, oregano, thyme, garlic, salt, paprika, and cayenne pepper and mix.

2. Put in the chicken fillets and allow them to marinate in the spices for preferable in a fridge overnight or for 30 minutes.

3. To prepare the coat, crack the egg in a bowl, add in the sriracha, cream, and Dijon mustard then mix.

4. Put the whey protein powder in a third bowl and set aside.

5. Now, drench the chicken pieces in the egg mixture and then dip in the whey protein powder to coat evenly.

6. Using a deep pan, pour in your oil of choice enough to submerge 4 chicken fillets at a go.

7. Bring the oil to heat over medium to high heat before frying the chicken pieces till cooked through and golden. This should take roughly 5 minutes per batch.

8. You will know the chicken is cooked through if the internal temperature gets to 75 °C/ 165 °F. Alternatively, cut open to test.

9. Serve immediately to enjoy the crispy exterior coat.

Pan-Seared Salmon with Chunky Avocado Salad

Time: 20 minutes | Servings 1

Kcal 847, Carbs 8.9g/0.31oz, Fats 64.2g/2.26oz, Proteins 49.4g/1.74oz, Fiber 14.3g/0.5oz

Ingredients:

Avocado salad

- 🍽 Pepper and sea salt

- 🍽 1 large diced avocado

- 🍽 15ml/1 tablespoon of extra virgin olive oil

- 🍽 ½ diced red onions

- 🍽 30ml/2 tablespoons of fresh lime juice

Salmon

- 🍽 7.5ml/½ a tablespoon of ghee or avocado oil

- 🍽 225g/0.5 lb salmon steak

- 🍽 Pepper and sea salt

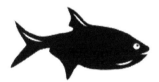

Instructions:

1. Halve, pit, and dice the avocado in a large bowl. Marsh half of the avocado dices using a fork.

2. Put in the remainder of the avocado sliced, diced red onions, olive oil, pepper, salt, and lime juice.

3. Combine thoroughly and put away in a fridge.

4. Add some pepper and salt to the salmon (sliced either large or small pieces depending on your preference).

5. Using a cast-iron skillet, bring the avocado oil to heat before searing the seasoned salmon of 5 minutes until it releases easily from the bottom.

6. Turn over to the other side and sear for an additional 5 minutes till both sides are brown and release easily from the pan. (Note that searing time will be relative depending on the size of the salmon pieces.)

7. Serve the salmon with the avocado salad on the side. Drizzle with extra lime juice if you so wish.

Keto Spicy Chicken Satay

Time: 20 minutes | Servings 2

Kcal 545, Carbs 9g/0.31oz, Fats 35g/1.23oz, Proteins 45.4g/1.6oz, Fiber 7.1g/o.25oz

Ingredients:

- 200g/7oz broccoli florets or broccolini

- 300g/10.6oz chicken breast slices

- 30ml/2 tablespoons of water

- Pepper and sea salt

- 10ml/2 teaspoons of sriracha hot sauce

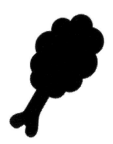

- 15ml/1 tablespoon of avocado oil or ghee

- 83g/3oz of almond or peanut butter

- 2 teaspoons of coconut aminos

Instructions:

1. Chop chicken breasts into smaller slices before adding some pepper and salt.

2. Put some water to boil in a pot.

3. Using either a griddle pan or a frying pan, grease the insides with generous amounts of ghee.

4. Arrange the chicken tender pieces on the pre-oiled pan and let them cook for 10 minutes turning halfway through.

5. In a mixing bowl, combine sriracha, almond butter, and coconut aminos before mixing carefully. Add some water to the mixture and mix some more till you achieve a smooth consistency.

6. Put all the broccoli in a steamer basket and steam over the boiling water till just tender.

7. Pour ⅓ of the sriracha sauce on the chicken tender pieces and coat evenly.

8. Serve the chicken with tenders with the steamed broccoli on the sides.

9. Top with the remainder of the sriracha sauce if desired.

Keto Shrimp Meygoo Polo

Time: 30 minutes | Servings 4

Kcal 386, Carbs 7.8g/0.28oz, Fats 30g/1.05oz, Proteins 19.8g/0.7oz, Fiber 3.9g/0.14oz

Ingredients:

- 🍽 60ml/4 tablespoons of extra virgin olive oil
- 🍽 1 (620g/1.4 lb) medium cauliflower
- 🍽 1g/¼ teaspoon of cayenne
- 🍽 60ml/4 tablespoons of divided avocado oil or ghee
- 🍽 4g/1 teaspoon of ground cumin
- 🍽 15ml/1 tablespoon of white vinegar
- 🍽 4g/1 teaspoon of ground turmeric
- 🍽 Black pepper and sea salt
- 🍽 4g/1 teaspoon of unsweetened tomato paste
- 🍽 1 finely chopped small yellow onion
- 🍽 450g/1 lb of peeled and deveined shrimp

- 🍽 4 cloves of minced garlic
- 🍽 10g/½ a cup of fresh cilantro
- 🍽 4g/ ¼ a teaspoon of saffron and ground ginger

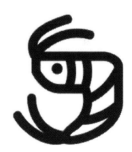

Instructions:

1. Make cauliflower rice by placing the cauliflower into a food processor Using the grating blade, shred the cauliflower into small rice-like pieces.

2. Generously grease the cooking surface of a large pan with ghee.

3. Put in the cauliflower rice and add some white vinegar and sauté for 5 minutes before seasoning with pepper and salt.

4. Move the sautéed cauliflower into a plate and set aside.

5. Using the same pan, add in the remainder of the ghee before pouring in the onion.

6. Cook until golden brown before adding in the garlic and let them cook for an additional minute.

7. Throw in the cayenne pepper, turmeric, tomato sauce, and salt. Fix everything up before adding saffron and ground ginger.

8. Now, put in the shrimp and cook together till the shrimp is cooked through roughly for around 3 minutes then top with the cilantro.

9. On a serving plate, serve some cauliflower rice and add the shrimp atop.

10. Spread some olive oil atop.

11. Enjoy!

12. If you wish to store, allow the meal to cool before refrigerating for up to 3 days.

Low-Carb Ginger Pork Cauliflower Rice Bowl

Time: 25 minutes | Servings 3
Kcal 428, Carbs 8.7g/0.3oz, Fats 29.4g/1.04oz, Proteins 31.5g/1.11oz, Fiber 3.6g/0.12oz

Ingredients:

- 45ml/3 tablespoons of extra virgin olive oil
- 400g/14.1oz cauliflower florets, riced
- 1 thinly sliced medium green onion
- 30ml/2 tablespoons of avocado oil or ghee
- 30g/2 tablespoons of chopped mint
- A pinch of ground black pepper
- ½ a medium cucumber
- 400g/14.1oz of ground pork (10% fat)
- 15g/¼ cup of chopped cilantro
- A pinch of sea salt
- 2 cloves of minced garlic

- 30ml/2 tablespoons of coconut aminos or tamari sauce
- 1 chopped medium mild chile pepper
- 45ml/3 tablespoons of divided lime juice
- 18 g/0.6oz of grated fresh ginger

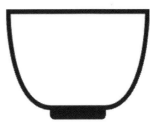

Instructions:

1. Put all the cauliflower rice in a food processor and pulse using the shredding blade into a small rice consistency.

2. Put the avocado oil or ghee on a frying pan. Add in the cauliflower rice and cook under medium heat for 6 minutes till cooked through.

3. Add some pepper and salt before transferring to a separate bowl and set it aside.

4. Using the same skillet, throw in the pork and fry till cooked for roughly 7 minutes.

5. Put in the mild chile pepper, ginger, and garlic. Combine and cook for a minute till nice and fragrant.

6. Once cooked, remove from the heat and pour in some lime juice and some coconut aminos and finally stir in the cilantro.

7. In a separate smaller bowl, mix the remainder of the lime juice and coconut aminos.

8. Chop the cucumber into smaller chunks and toss the amino mix through before stirring through with the coriander and mint.

9. On a serving plate, first, serve the cauliflower rice and ground pork on top.

10. Garnish with mint and chopped green onions.

11. Finish off with a drizzle of extra virgin olive oil atop.

Keto Spiced Cauliflower Rice with Sardines

Time: 25 minutes | Servings 4

Kcal 433, Carbs 9.6g/0.33oz, Fats 31.3g/1.1oz, Proteins 25.7g/0.9oz, Fiber 5.4g/0.19oz

Ingredients:

- 340g/12oz of drained canned sardines in spring water or olive oil
- 600g/1.3 lbs of cauliflower cut into florets
- 30ml/2 tablespoons of fresh lime juice
- 90ml/4 tablespoons of extra virgin olive oil
- 30g/2 tablespoons of chopped fresh cilantro
- ½ diced red bell pepper
- 60ml/¼ cup of water or chicken stock
- ½ diced green bell pepper
- 240ml/1 cup of tomato sauce
- ½ diced small red onion
- Black pepper and sea salt

- 2g/½ a teaspoon of garlic powder
- 1g/¼ teaspoon of chili powder
- 8g/2 teaspoons of smoked or sweet paprika
- 4g/1 teaspoon of dried oregano
- 4g/1 teaspoon of dried cumin

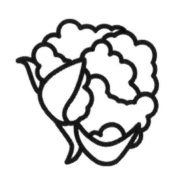

Instructions:

1. Reduce the cauliflower into florets before pulsing in a food processor til small rice sized consistency.

2. Bring 30ml/2 tablespoons of oil to heat on a pan over medium to low heat and put in the diced onion and the capsicums.

3. Now quickly fry the vegetable mixture before adding in the dried herbs and sauté some more till nice and fragrant.

4. Pour in the chicken stock and tomato sauce and bring the mixture to simmer.

5. Reduce the heat before putting in the cauliflower rice and mix everything up.

6. Stir continuously while the cauliflower is cooking adding in the seasoning accordingly.

7. When cooked, add in half the cilantro and stir.

8. Serve the rice into 4 plates, top with sardines, chili slices, fresh lime wedges and coriander leaves.

9. Finish off with a drizzle of olive oil atop.

Chops with Green Beans and Avocado

Time: 55 minutes | Serves 4
Kcal 887, Carbs 6g/0.21oz, Fat 76g/2.68oz, Protein 39g/1.38oz, Fiber 9g/0.32oz

ngredients:

- 🍽 Pepper

- 🍽 6 scallions

- 🍽 2 avocados

- 🍽 8g/2 teaspoons of salt

- 🍽 8g/2 teaspoon of ground
  black pepper

- 🍽 60ml/4 tablespoon of olive oil

- 🍽 900g/2⁄3 lb of green beans

- 🍽 113g/4oz butter

- 🍽 1g/¼ teaspoon of paprika

- 🍽 1 clove of garlic

- 🍽 4 pork shoulder chops

- 🍽 30ml/2 tablespoon
  mild chipotle paste

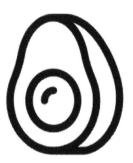

Instructions:

1. Prepare a mixture of oil, salt, and chipotle paste

2. Smear the meat with the marinade and let it sit for 15 minutes. If you have more time to spare, marinate the meat in a plastic bag in the refrigerator.

3. Bring the oven to heat up to 200 °C/ 400 °F.

4. Place the marinated meat in the oven and let it cook for 30 minutes until nice and ready. Remember to turn the meat every 10 minutes for even cooking.

5. As the meat is cooking, crush the clove of garlic, mix with spices and butter then put it aside.

6. On a frying pan, sauté the beans slowly on medium heat until they get that nice color. Reduce the heat when almost cooked and add the spices.

7. Finally, peel and mash the avocado then mix it with finely chopped onion rings. Combine the avocado and onion mash with the cooked beans and season with salt and pepper.

8. Serve with baked pork and some chopped cilantro to your liking.

Keto Mackerel Patties

Time: 20 minutes | Servings 9 patties
Kcal 486, Carbs 2.9g/0.1oz, Fats 34.8g/1.22oz, Proteins 37.8g/1.33oz, Fiber 2.4g/0.08oz

Ingredients:

- 15ml/1 teaspoon of extra virgin avocado oil or ghee
- 400g/14.1oz canned and drained mackerel
- A pinch of pepper
- A pinch of sea salt
- 4g/1 teaspoon of onion powder
- 15g/1 tablespoon of chopped parsley
- 60g/2.1oz of almond flour
- 15ml/1 tablespoon of Dijon mustard
- 1 large egg
- 15ml/1 tablespoon of paleo mayonnaise

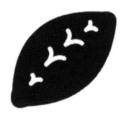

Instructions:

1. Put the mackerel in a mixing bowl and mash using a fork.

2. Add in all ingredients, olive oil, and ¼ a cup of almond flour to the mashed mackerel and mix thoroughly.

3. Make 9 patties using your hands then flatten them using the palms of your hand before dusting each patty with the remainder of the almond flour.

4. Add the ghee in a frying pan before bringing it to heat over medium heat.

5. Cook the patties for 8 minutes flipping halfway through to brown both sides.

6. Enjoy with a beverage of your choice.

7. You can store the cooked patties in a refrigerator for 4 days. Be sure to reheat before serving.

Dinner Recipes

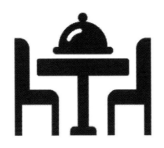

Low-Carb Chicken Fajita Dinner Bowl

Time: 30 minutes | Servings 4
Kcal 602, Carbs 8.8g/0.31oz, Fats 46.6g/1.64oz, Proteins 32.9g/1.16oz, Fiber 6.8g/0.24oz

Ingredients:

- 60ml/4 tablespoons of extra virgin olive oil
- 500g/1.1 lb (2) skinless chicken breasts
- 4 sprigs fresh cilantro
- 30g/2 tablespoons of taco seasoning
- 340ml/1 cup of sour cream
- 45ml/3 tablespoons of extra virgin avocado oil
- 120g/4 cups of baby spinach leaves
- 1 medium red pepper
- 1 medium green pepper
- 1 medium yellow pepper
- 1 large avocado
- ½ small red onion

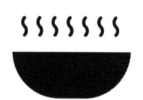

Instructions:

1. Begin by assembling all the necessary ingredients.

2. Arrange the chicken breasts on a baking sheet before coating with some avocado oil. Go ahead and apply 1 tablespoon of seasoning rub on each side.

3. Using your hands, massage in the rub before searing the breasts on a BBQ or grill plate till nice and caramelized.

4. Now, reduce the heat to a medium or low and cook further till all the fluid drains completely.

5. Remove from the source of heat and wrap with a foil then set aside.

6. Clean, peel, and dice the red onion into a bowl.

7. Clean, deseed, and chop the peppers into coarse strips.

8. On a large skillet, bring 1 tablespoon of olive oil to heat up and cook the onions and peppers till nice and tender.

9. Unravel the foil, and slice the chicken breast into thin strips across the grain.

10. Arrange the bowl having the spinach at the bottom, followed by roasted veggies, and chicken strips. Finish off with sour cream and avocado atop.

11. Sprinkle with coriander and olive oil for garnish.

12. For storage, put it into a sealed package and refrigerate for 3 days or less. If you intend to store, don't include the avocado, rather preserve and cut it fresh when you are ready to consume.

Mexican Keto Empanadas

Time: 50 minutes | Servings 12 empanadas
Kcal 346, Carbs 5.2g/0.18oz, Fats 27.1g/0.96oz, Proteins 20.1g/0.71oz, Fiber 2.6g/0.09oz

Ingredients:

For the filling

- 1 large beaten egg
- 15ml/1 tablespoon of extra virgin olive oil
- 120ml/½ a cup of chicken stock or bone broth
- 500g/1.1 lb of ground beef
- 15ml/1 tablespoon of coconut aminos
- 1 small chopped yellow onion
- 15ml/1 tablespoon of unsweetened tomato paste
- 1 small chopped red bell pepper
- 15ml/1 tablespoon of taco seasoning
- 1 chopped small green bell pepper
- 250g/8.8oz diced radishes

For the pasty

- 2g/½ a teaspoon of ground black pepper
- 340g/3 cups of low moisture shredded mozzarella cheese
- A pinch of salt
- 75g/5 tablespoons of cream cheese
- 4g/1 teaspoon of onion powder
- 2 large eggs
- 4g/1 teaspoon of garlic powder
- 200g/2 cups of almond flour

Instructions:

1. Using a large skillet, bring the oil to heat then add in the garlic and onion.

2. Cook till onions begin to brown before adding in the ground beef, cook some more till the beef gets nice and brown.

3. Put in the diced capsicums and radishes. Cook until the veggies get tender for roughly 10 minutes.

4. Now pour in the chicken stock, taco seasoning, coconut aminos, and tomato paste, stir in well.

5. Let the mixture simmer till the chicken stock absorbs into the mixture before removing it from the heat.

6. Bring the oven to a temperature of 190 °C/ 375 °F.

7. Using a microwavable bowl, combine the cream cheese and mozzarella then heat for 2 minutes stirring midway through.

8. Now, to the mozzarella and cream mix, add the 2 beaten eggs, almond flour, and seasonings. Mix till you achieve an even dough.

9. Divide the dough evenly into 12 circular pieces

10. Lay 2 grease-proof papers on a tough working surface and roll each piece of dough into thin flat rounds.

11. Scoop and place a spoonful of the prepared filling at the center.

12. Crack and whisk the remaining egg into a consistent wash. Coat the margins/edges of the dough before folding and scaling using your hands.

13. Line a baking sheet with parchment paper before carefully arranging the empanadas.

14. Brush the surface with the egg wash before baking in the oven for 20 minutes.

15. Serve with sour cream for dipping.

Keto Ham and Cheese Chaffle Sandwich

Time: 15 minutes | Servings 2
Kcal 733, Carbs 8.4g/0.29oz, Fats 57.1g/2.01oz, Proteins 45.8g/1.62oz, Fiber 3.3g/0.12oz

Ingredients:

For the chaffles

- 1g/¼ a teaspoon of gluten-free baking powder
- 1 large egg

For the filling

- 2 small lettuce leaves
- 2 slices (46g/1.6oz) of ham
- 4 slices of tomato

- 25g/¼ cup of almond flour
- 57g/½ a cup of shredded cheddar cheese

Instructions:

1. Combine all the chaffle ingredients in a mixing bowl and stir thoroughly till even.

2. Scoop half of the mixture and put it into a hot waffle maker to make a single waffle.

3. Close the waffle maker and allow cooking for 4 minutes.

4. Open the lid when done and allow the waffle to cool down before moving the chaffle to cool further.

5. Repeat the same procedure for the remainder of the batter.

6. Allow the chaffles to cool down entirely for that crisp finish.

7. Now arrange to have a slice of chaffle at the bottom followed with ham, cheese, tomato, and finally lettuce before covering with another chaffle slice.

8. Enjoy!

9. Store the chaffles in a closed package for 3 days or in a fridge for a whole week. Remember don't store with the toppings.

Seared Pork Chops with Creamy Cheese Sauce

Time: 45 minutes | Servings 4
Kcal 446, Carbs 3.9g/0.13oz, Fats 34.6g/1.22oz, Proteins 28.5g/1oz, Fiber 0.7g/0.02oz

ngredients:

- 56g/½ a cup of shredded mozzarella cheese
- 450g/1 lb pork loin chops
- 30g/2 tablespoons of fresh thyme
- 15ml/1 tablespoon of extra virgin olive oil
- 60ml/¼ cup of heavy whipping cream
- Black pepper and sea salt
- 1 clove of minced garlic
- 2 medium yellow onions
- 360ml/1½ beef stock
- 57g/½ stick butter

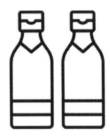

Instructions:

1. Pat the pork chops till dry before adding some pepper and salt to taste.

2. Using a large pan, bring the olive oil to heat under medium temperature. Fry the pork chops till brown and crispy for 8 minutes flipping them halfway through.

3. Transfer to a separate bowl when cooked.

4. Using the same pan, melt the butter before adding in thinly sliced onions.

5. Sauté them over medium to high heat till nice and caramelized.

6. Now, add in garlic, pepper, salt, and the beef stock and allow the mixture to simmer till the broth reduces and thickens. Finish off with some cream then stir.

7. Dip the pork chop pieces into the broth and let everything simmer for an additional 10 minutes.

8. Spread the mozzarella cheese atop and cover the pan. Cook until all the cheese melts.

9. Serve with some thyme sprigs garnish.

Keto Cheese Stuffed Crust Pizza

Time: 30 minutes | Servings 1 pizza 8 slices
Kcal 262, Carbs 4.5g/0.16oz, Fats 19.2g/0.68oz, Proteins 17.6g/0.62oz, Fiber 1.1g/0.03oz

Ingredients:

For the crust

- 150g/5.3oz of string cheese sticks
- 170g/1½ cup of shredded mozzarella
- 67g/⅔ cup of almond flour

For the topping

- Black pepper
- 125g/½ a cup of tomato passata
- 150g/5.3oz of mozzarella slices
- ¼ cup of thinly sliced basil

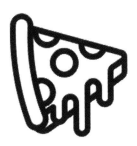

Instructions:

1. Bring the oven to a temperature of 200 °C/ 400 °F.

2. Place the shredded mozzarella into a microwavable dish and melt for minute before stirring and melting once more till it is completely melted

3. Combine with almond flour and mix to a dough.

4. Roll the dough to a larger circle than needed for the pizza.

5. Arrange the cheese sticks around the edges of the circular flattened dough and roll the edge over to hold the cheese sticks in place.

6. Lay a baking tray with parchment paper and transfer and put the dough on top. Cook in the oven for 10 minutes till cooked.

7. Once cooked, lay out the passata on the pizza crust and top with shredded mozzarella cheese.

8. Cover with the mozzarella slices before baking further in the oven for 1 minutes.

9. Garnish with shredded basil and black pepper.

10. Finish off with a drizzle of olive oil and enjoy!

Chicken Wings with Creamy Broccoli

Time: 55 minutes | Serves 4

Kcal 1215, Carbs 9g/0.31oz, Fats 100g/3.5oz, Protein 65g/2.3oz, Fiber 5g/0.17oz

ngredients:

- 🍽 Broccoli

- 🍽 Salt and pepper

- 🍽 1 cup mayo

- 🍽 ½ cup chopped dill

- 🍽 680g/1½ lbs broccoli

- 🍽 Chicken wings

- 🍽 1.3kg/3 lbs chicken

- 🍽 A pinch of salt

- 🍽 2g/½ teaspoon cayenne pepper

- 🍽 ¼ cup olive oil

- 🍽 8g/2 teaspoon ground ginger

- 🍽 1 orange, juice, and zest

Instructions:

1. Bring the oven to heat up to 200 °C/ 400 °F.

2. Juice the orange, mix the juice and zest with other spices and olive oil.

3. Put the chicken wings in a plastic bag and empty the marinade into the bag.

4. Shake and mix up the wings with the mixture and allow it to settle and marinate for five minutes or more.

5. After marinating, place the wings in a greased baking dish before throwing them in a rack or broiler for that extra crisp finish.

6. Cook in the oven until the wings are nice and brown. This should take around 45 minutes to achieve.

7. While the wings are cooking, chop the broccoli into florets and partially boil in salted water for a few minutes until they soften but not lose their shape.

8. Strain and allow the broccoli to release steam before adding the rest of the ingredients.

9. Serve with the cooked wings and enjoy!

Prosciutto Wrapped Halloumi

Time: 20 minutes | Servings 2

Kcal 476, Carbs 2.5g/0.09oz, Fats 37.2g/1.31oz, Proteins 32.7g/1.15oz, Fiber 0

Ingredients:

- 🍴 60g/2.1oz (4 slices) prosciutto di Parma
- 🍴 250g/8.8oz halloumi cheese (chopped into 8 sticks)

Instructions:

1. Bring the oven to a temperature of 240 °C/ 465 °F then line the baking tray with parchment paper.

2. Chop the halloumi cheese into 8 equal pieces and the prosciutto into long halfways.

3. On every stick wrap with a slice of ham.

4. Place on the tray having the seam side facing downwards. Cook in the oven for approximately 15 minutes flipping midway through.

5. Serve while warm with some BBQ sauce or low carb ketchup.

Pan-Fried Sea Bass with Butter Samphire

Time: 10 minutes | Servings 1

Kcal 550, Carbs 2.3g/0.08oz, Fats 43.6g/1.54oz, Proteins 34.2g/1.2oz, Fiber 5.1g/0.18oz

Ingredients:

- 15ml/1 tablespoon of fresh lemon juice
- 2 fillets (150g/7oz) of sea bass or trout
- 100g/3.5oz samphire or spinach
- 15ml/1 tablespoons of avocado oil or ghee
- A pinch of pepper
- 28g/2 tablespoons of unsalted butter or ghee
- A pinch of salt

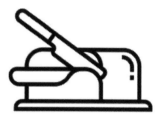

Instructions:

1. On a flat plate lay the sea bass or trout fillets before sea pepper and salt.

2. Grease a skillet with avocado oil and bring it to heat. Now, lay the sea bass skin side facing down and cook till nice and crispy for 4 minutes.

3. Turn on the other side using a spatula and allow cooking for an additional 3 to 4 minutes.

4. Once done, remove from heat and put aside.

5. Using the same skillet, add in the butter before putting the samphire or spinach. Don't add salt if you are using the samphire, it is naturally salty.

6. Sauté for 3 minutes tossing frequently for an even finish.

7. To serve begin with the samphire and lay the sea bass on top.

8. Sprinkle the lemon juice atop and enjoy while warm.

Keto Teriyaki Chicken Bowl

Time: 30 minutes | Servings 1
Kcal 587, Carbs 9g/0.32oz, Fats 45.2g/1.59oz, Proteins 33.8g/1.19oz, Fiber 4.2g/0.14oz

Ingredients:

For the chicken

- 15ml/1 tablespoon of ghee
- 140g/6oz diced chicken thighs
- 1g/¼ teaspoon of garlic powder
- 18g/1 tablespoon of tamari sauce
- 1g/¼ teaspoon of ground ginger
- 10g/1 tablespoon of Erythritol

For the veggies

- 1 thinly sliced onion
- 75g/3.5oz medium diced zucchini
- ¼ diced small yellow onion
- ½ a cup of steamed broccoli
- 30g/2 tablespoons of ghee
- 60g/½ a cup of cauliflower rice
- Sea salt
- 2g/½ a teaspoon of sesame seeds

Instructions:

1. Using a good-sized bowl, add in all the ingredients for preparing the chicken and mix everything up.

2. Now, toss in the diced chicken pieces and allow to marinate overnight or 30 minutes in the refrigerator.

3. Bring a skillet to heat over medium to high temperatures before putting in the marinated chicken.

4. Cook the chicken dices for 4 minutes per side till nice and brown then remove and put aside.

5. Using the same pan, put in the butter and sauté the onions and zucchini for 3 minutes till nice and tender. Put in the sesame seeds and mix.

6. To serve, put the cauliflower rice on one ¼ of the plate, steamed broccoli to another ¼, chicken on the third ¼, and finally the veggies on the last ¼ of the plate.

Low-Carb Broccoli Cheese Gratin

Time: 50 minutes | Servings 4

Kcal 263, Carbs 6.7g/0.24oz, Fats 21.9g/0.77oz, Proteins 11.5g/0.4oz, Fiber 3.4g/0.12oz

Ingredients:

- 🍽 113g/1 cup of grated cheddar cheese

- 🍽 450g/1 lb broccoli

- 🍽 2g/½ a teaspoon of ground black pepper

- 🍽 2g/½ a teaspoon of garlic powder

- 🍽 A pinch of sea salt

- 🍽 28g/2 tablespoons of unsalted butter

- 🍽 240ml/1 cup of unsweetened almond milk

- 🍽 1g/¼ teaspoon of xanthan gum

- 🍽 80g/⅓ cup of cream cheese

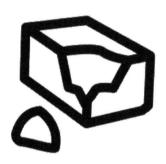

Instructions:

1. Bring the oven to a temperature of 200 °C/ 400 °F.

2. Steam the broccoli until just tender enough on the inside.

3. Lightly oil a casserole dish and put in the steamed broccoli.

4. Using a small saucepan, melt in the butter and add in the xanthan gum then mix.

5. Now, add in the cream cheese, almond milk, and garlic powder and continue stirring till you achieve an even sauce.

6. Remove from the heat when done and add in some cheddar cheese before pouring over the broccoli.

7. Stir everything gently and add the remainder of the cheddar cheese atop.

8. Cook in the pre-heated oven till all the cheese melts and browns at the top.

9. Serve and enjoy immediately.

Quick Keto Snack Recipes

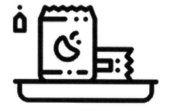

Kale Chips

Time: 25 minutes | Serving 4

Kcal 58, Carbs 3g/0.1oz, Fats 4g/0.14oz, Protein 2g/0.07oz, Fiber 2g/0.07oz

Ingredients:

- Salt
- 5ml/½ a teaspoon lemon juice
- 226g/½ lb kale
- 15ml/1 tablespoon olive oil

Instructions:

1. Bring the oven to a temperature of 150 °C/300 °F.

2. Remove the stalk and reduce the leaves to smaller pieces.

3. Immerse the kale in olive oil and lemon juice and season with some salt.

4. Bake for 15 minutes till crispy.

Low-Carb Spinach Artichoke Bacon Cups

Time: 40 minutes | Servings 12 cups
Kcal 200, Carbs 3.2g/0.11oz, Fats 17.3g/0.61oz, Proteins 9.5g/0.34oz, Fiber 1.3g/0.05oz

Ingredients:

- 🍽 360g/13oz streaky bacon cut into 24 thin slices

- 🍽 240g/8.5oz artichokes hearts (1 can)

- 🍽 45g/1½ cups of freshly chopped spinach

- 🍽 ½ minced yellow onion

- 🍽 Black pepper and sea salt

- 🍽 113g/1 cup of mozzarella cheese(shredded)

- 🍽 2 cloves of minced garlic

- 🍽 227g/8oz of cream cheese

- 🍽 30g/⅓ cup of grated Parmesan cheese

- 🍽 115g/½ cup of sour cream

nstructions:

1. Bring the oven to a temperature of 200 °C/ 400 °F.

2. Put the artichoke hearts into a mixing bowl.

3. Add in every other ingredient but the bacon then mix everything till well combined.

4. Using a 12-cup muffin pan, wrap a slice of bacon against the wall of a cup and cut a slice into 2, arrange the pieces at the bottom to cover the entire cup with bacon strips.

5. Do the same for the rest of the cups. (2 bacon strips per cup).

6. Scoop the artichoke mixture and put it into each cup lined with bacon.

7. Cook in the oven till the bacon turns brown and crisp while the mix melts. Let the bacon cups cool before removing from the muffin tray.

8. Serve and enjoy!

Keto Caramelized Pecans

Time: 20 minutes | Servings 8

Kcal 193, Carbs 1.2g/0.04oz, Fats 20.1g/0.71oz, Proteins 2.3g/0.08oz, Fiber 2.4g/0.084oz

Ingredients:

- 200g/2 cups of pecan halves
- 1g/¼ teaspoon of cinnamon
- 4g/1 teaspoon of sugar-free maple extract
- 4g/1 teaspoon of sugar-free vanilla extract
- 20ml/4 teaspoons of virgin coconut oil or ghee
- 30g/2 tablespoons of low-carb sweetener
- A pinch of salt

Instructions:

1. Bring the oven to a temperature of 170 °C/ 340 °F.
2. Combine all the dry ingredients in a bowl and mix thoroughly.
3. In a separate bowl, mix the oil and with the maple extract.
4. Line the baking tray with parchment paper and spread the nuts evenly.
5. Coat with some oil evenly before dusting over the nuts with the dry and sweetener.
6. Cook for 15 minutes in the oven tossing halfway through.
7. Once done, remove from the oven and allow cooling for 5 minutes.
8. Enjoy it when cool and crispy!

Meal Prep Special for 7 Days

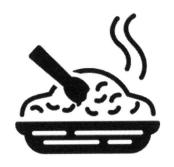

Day 1

Breakfast: Full English Keto Breakfast

Time: 15 minutes | Servings 1
Kcal 658, Carbs 7g/0.25oz, Fats 55g/1.94oz, Proteins 29.6g/1.04oz, Fiber 8.3g/0.29oz

Ingredients:

- Pepper and salt
- 15ml/1 tablespoon of ghee
- ½ sliced avocado
- 5 brown mushrooms
- 5 cherry tomatoes
- 75g/2.7oz bacon sliced into 6 thin pieces
- 78g/2.8oz frozen spinach (drained and thawed.)
- 2 large eggs
- 15ml/1 tablespoon of olive oil

1. Grease a good-sized pan with ghee and bring to heat over medium to high temperature.

2. Season the mushroom with pepper and salt before frying in the pan having the top side facing downwards.

3. Let the mushrooms cook for 5 minutes before flipping and cooking for 2 more minutes then move to a plate.

4. In a different skillet, fry the bacon pieces till crispy on both sides and set aside.

5. Now fry the eggs, using the same skillet you cooked the bacon in until the egg whites begin to set but the yolk is still runny.

6. Continuing with the same skillet, put in the cherry tomatoes and fry for a minute.

7. Drain water from the spinach before serving.

8. Now, serve everything on a plate with sliced avocado on the side. Top with olive oil and enjoy!

Lunch: Low-Carb Palmini Spaghetti Bolognese (See page 48)

Dinner: Low-Carb Chicken Fajita Dinner Bowl (See page 68)

Day 2

Breakfast: Keto Feta Quiche and Spinach (See page 27)

Lunch: Creamy Low-Carb Chicken with Capers
Time: 25 minutes | Servings 2
Kcal 574, Carbs 8.8g/0.31oz, Fats 44.6g/1.57oz, Proteins 41.1g/1.45oz, Fiber 2.7g/0.09oz

Ingredients:

- 🍽 180g/¾ block of soft cream cheese
- 🍽 340g/12oz skinless and boneless chicken thighs
- 🍽 17g/2 tablespoons capers
- 🍽 Pepper and salt
- 🍽 30ml/2 tablespoons of lemon juice
- 🍽 30ml/2 tablespoons of extra virgin olive oil
- 🍽 120g/1 cup frozen green beans
- 🍽 1 clove of minced garlic
- 🍽 4g/1 teaspoon of dried Italian herbs
- 🍽 8g/2 teaspoons of onion powder

Instructions:

1. Collect and assemble all the ingredients.

2. Slice the chicken thighs into small bite-size pieces before adding pepper and salt to taste.

3. Bring the oil to heat in the skillet and brown the chicken pieces. Pour in the lemon juice and seasoning then stir.

4. Put in the capers and green beans and mix well.

5. Let everything cook for 5 minutes before adding the cream cheese in tiny chunks. Stir continuously as you add in the cream cheese until fully melted and covering the rest of the dish.

6. Serve and enjoy.

Dinner: Mexican Keto Empanadas (See page 70)

Day 3

Breakfast: Keto Single-Serve Peach Cobbler (See page 29)

Lunch: Keto Chicken Spinach and Artichoke Casserole (See page 49)

Dinner: Low-Carb Chicken Parmesan Skillet
Time: 20 minutes | Servings 2
Kcal 524, Carbs 6.5g/0.22oz, Fats 35.6g/1.25oz, Proteins 42g/1.48oz, Fiber 1.8g/0.06oz

Ingredients:

- 🍽 2g/½ a teaspoon of Italian dry herbs

- 🍽 300g/10.6oz, 2 medium skinless and boneless chicken breasts

- 🍽 30g/4 tablespoons of grated Parmesan cheese

- 🍽 15ml/1 tablespoon of extra virgin olive oil

- 🍽 28g/¼ cup of grated mozzarella cheese

- 🍽 240ml/1 cup of sugar-free marinara sauce

Instructions:

1. Bring the top element of the oven to a temperature of 200 °C/ 400 °F.

2. In a skillet, bring the olive oil to heat under medium to high-temperature setting then cook the breast for 10 minutes flipping halfway through.

3. Now, pour the marinara sauce around the cooked chicken, then add in the herbs.

4. Cook everything in the oven till the chicken is nice and golden and the cheese is fully melted.

5. Serve with steamed veggies on the side.

Day 4

Breakfast: Almond Flour Keto Muffins

Time: 20 minutes | Servings 12 muffins

Kcal 191, Carbs 2.6g/0.09oz, Fats 17.4g/0.61oz, Proteins 6.1g/0.21oz, Fiber 2.1g/0.07oz

Ingredients:

- 🍽 5ml/1 teaspoon of sugar-free vanilla extract

- 🍽 250g/2½ cups of almond flour

- 🍽 160ml/⅔ cup of unsweetened almond milk

- 🍽 135g/⅔ cup granulated Erythritol

- 🍽 3 lightly beaten eggs

- 🍽 80ml/⅓ cup unsalted melted butter

Instructions:

1. Bring the oven to a temperature of 180 °C/ 355 °F.

2. Put all the dry ingredients in a mixing bowl then mix thoroughly.

3. In a separate bowl, combine almond milk, eggs, melted butter, and vanilla and mix well.

4. Now combine with the dry ingredients.

5. Using a 12-cup silicone muffin divided the mixture equally into the cups and be sure not to fill to the brim.

6. In the oven, cook for 25 minutes until cooked through. Insert a skewer to check readiness, if it comes out clean then it is ready.

7. Allow the muffins to cool before serving with a sugar-free beverage of your choice.

Lunch: Low-Carb Crispy Fried KFC Chicken (See page 51)

Dinner: Keto Ham and Cheese Chaffle Sandwich (See page 73)

Day 5

Breakfast: Spinach and Feta ShakShuka (See page 31)

Lunch: Keto Soul Food Chicken Meatball Soup

Time: 25 minutes | Servings 4

Kcal 334, Carbs 6.1g/0.22oz, Fats 19.2g/0.68oz, Proteins 32.1g/1.13oz, Fiber 2.5g/0.09oz

Ingredients:

For the meatballs

- 🍽 15ml/1 tablespoon ghee
- 🍽 450g/1 lb, 2 chicken breast pieces
- 🍽 1g/¼ a teaspoon of cracked black pepper
- 🍽 ½ brown onion cut into wedges

- 🍽 A pinch of salt
- 🍽 2 roughly chopped cloves of garli
- 🍽 25g/2 tablespoons of chopped parsley
- 🍽 15g/1 tablespoon of tomato pure

For the soup

- 🍽 15g/1 tablespoon chopped parsley
- 🍽 30ml/2 tablespoons of coconut oil
- 🍽 100g/2 cups of chopped kale
- 🍽 ½ chopped brown onion
- 🍽 A pinch of cracked black pepper
- 🍽 2 medium chopped celery sticks
- 🍽 A pinch of sea salt
- 🍽 2 chopped medium carrots

- 🍽 4g/1 teaspoon dried thyme
- 🍽 1.5L/6 cups of chicken stock

Instructions:

1. Bring the oven to a temperature of 200 °C/ 390 °F.

2. Combine all the chicken meatball into a food processor and pulse to evenly mix.

3. Make 20 meatballs from the mixture by dividing and rolling with your hands.

4. Line the baking tray with parchment paper before arranging the meatballs and coating each one of them with melted ghee.

5. Cook in the oven till brown and cooked through for approximately 20 minutes.

6. While the meatballs are baking, put the butter in a skillet and melt under medium to low heat.

7. Now fry the celery, carrots, and onions for a few minutes until tender.

8. Pour in the thyme, chicken stock, and seasoning then stir.

9. Lower the heat and allow the mixture to simmer for roughly 10 minutes.

10. Throw in the kales and let them soften for 2 minutes before topping with the meatballs and adjusting the seasoning accordingly.

11. Finish off with the parsley to garnish.

12. Enjoy while warm.

Dinner: Seared Pork Chops with Creamy Cheese Sauce (See page 75)

Day 6

Breakfast: Keto Apricot Crumble Coffee Cake (See page 35)

Lunch: Keto Spicy Chicken Satay (See page 55)

Dinner: Coconut curry chicken

Time: 50 minutes | Serves 4

Kcal 793, Carbs 8g/0.28oz, Fats 70g/2.45oz, Protein 33g/1.16oz, Fiber 5g/0.17oz

Ingredients:

- 🍽 30ml/2 tablespoons coconut oil
- 🍽 2 stalk of lemongrass
- 🍽 1 leek
- 🍽 17g/1 tablespoon of curry powder
- 🍽 680g/1½ lbs of boneless chicken thigh
- 🍽 2 garlic cloves
- 🍽 1 lime
- 🍽 A thumb-sized ginger
- 🍽 1 sliced red bell pepper
- 🍽 ½ chopped red chili pepper
- 🍽 396g/14oz coconut cream

Instructions:

1. Cut the chicken into fairly large pieces.

2. Crush the rough lemongrass on a pestle.

3. In a skillet, warm the coconut oil.

4. Grate the ginger and fry with the crushed lemongrass and some curry.

5. Sauté half of the chicken until stripes turn golden then season with salt and pepper and set aside.

6. In the same manner, fry the rest of the chicken but this time use more curry.

7. Slice and sauté the leaks on the same pan with the rest of the vegetables and chopped garlic.

8. Now put the coconut cream and chicken and allow it to simmer for 10 minutes

9. Remove the lemongrass and top with some lime zest.

Day 7

Breakfast: Keto Veggie Loa

Time: 85 minutes | Servings 12 slices

Kcal 175, Carbs 3.8g/0.13oz, Fats 14.6g/0.51oz, Proteins 6.7g/0.24oz, Fiber 3g/0.1oz

Ingredients:

- 15g/2 tablespoons mix seeds
- 100g/1 cup of almond flour
- 8g/2 teaspoons of pink Himalayan salt
- 65g/½ cup of mixed seeds (flax, pumpkin, and sunflower)
- 8g/2 teaspoons of baking powder
- 40g/⅓ cup of coconut flour
- 8g/2 teaspoons ground cumin
- 8g/2 teaspoons of psyllium husks
- 4g/1 teaspoon of smoked paprika
- 1 320g/11.3oz grated zucchini
- 60ml/¼ cup of ghee or coconut oil
- 1 small grated carrot
- 4 large eggs
- 115g/4.1oz grated pumpkin

Instructions:

1. Bring the oven to a temperature of Heat oven to 170 °C/ 340 °F.

2. In a mixing bowl, combine and stir all the dry ingredients till even.

3. In a different bowl, put in the grated veggies, eggs, and ghee then mix everything thoroughly.

4. Now combine the dry mixture with the veggies and mix further. Don't worry if the mixture will be rather dry.

5. Using a loaf pan lined with parchment paper, release the mixture in and press down. Top with the mixed seeds.

6. Cook in the oven for up to 70 minutes checking with the skewer until it comes out clean.

7. Allow cooling for roughly 30 minutes in the pan before transferring to the cooling rack.

8. Slice and enjoy with a low-carb beverage of your choice.

Lunch: Keto Shrimp Meygoo Polo (See page 57)

Dinner: Keto Cheese Stuffed Crust Pizza (See page 77)

Disclaimer

The opinions and ideas of the author contained in this publication are designed to educat the reader in an informative and helpful manner. While we accept that the instructions wi not suit every reader, it is only to be expected that the recipes might not gel with everyon Use the book responsibly and at your own risk. This work with all its contents, does n guarantee correctness, completion, quality or correctness of the provided informatio Always check with your medical practitioner should you be unsure whether to follow a lo carb eating plan. Misinformation or misprints cannot be completely eliminated. Huma error is real!

Design: Oliviaprodesign

Picture: Kiian Oksana / www.shutterstock.com

Printed by Amazon Italia Logistica S.r.l.
Torrazza Piemonte (TO), Italy

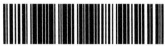